PREFACE

My name is Valencia Annik Payne M.S. Health Informatics/Healthcare Administration, Certificate Cyber Security, BSN RN, BS Biology. As the Author of Fluid and Electrolytes for Nursing Students, Dimensional Analysis for Nursing Students, GI for Nursing Students, Respiratory and Factures for Nursing Students, and now the arrival of Diabetes for Nursing Students is here! In the nursing profession, it not about learning one concept but all concepts as this will provide positive patient outcomes. Please enjoy this colorful and simplified learning tool.

© 2017 by Library of Congress. All rights reserved.
This book is protected by copyright. No part of it may be reproduced, stored in a retrieval system, or transmitted in any form or by any means: electronic, mechanical, photocopy, recording, or otherwise without prior written permission of the author.

ACKNOWLEDGEMENT

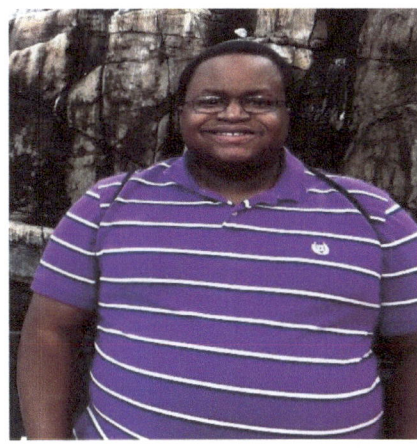

The cover illustrator is Mr. Hernando Cartes Payne II M.Ed., BS Biology. Mr. Payne has a natural talent for his intricate artwork. Mr. Payne teaches IPC and Principles of Engineering through Project Lead The Way in the Fort Bend Independent School District at Willowridge High School. Mr. Payne interest include Aerospace and General Science.

CONTENTS

Diabetes

Complications of Diabetes

DKA Treatment

Diabetes and Tooth Decay

What About My Thyroid?

Adrenal Cortex Issues

NCLEX Practice Question

NCLEX Answers

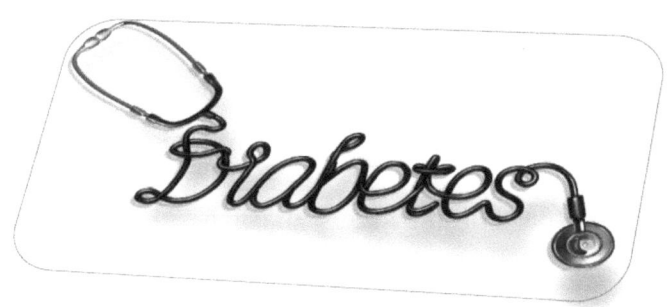

Diabetes is a condition in which the body does not process food properly in which to allow the body to have the proper energy needed to function. The food that we eat is turned into sugar or glucose for the body to use as energy. How is this possible is the pancreas makes and releases the hormone insulin to move the glucose from the bloodstream and into our cells for energy. The insulin also helps in regulating the body's blood glucose level.

TREATMENT OF DIABETES IN GENERAL

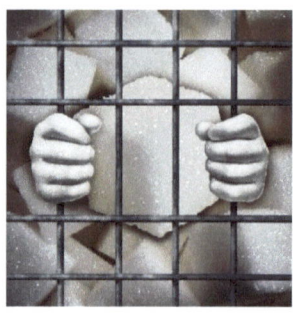

A. Exercise when the blood sugar is at its highest

B. Exercise at the same time and amount daily

C. Prior to exercise and to prevent hypoglycemia, please eat something

D. **Why are diabetics prone to coronary artery disease?** The sugar destroys blood vessels

E. A high fiber diet will keep the blood sugar steady (High fiber will slow down the absorption of glucose in the intestines, which eliminates the sharp fall and rise of the blood sugar)

F. Oral hypoglycemic stimulate the pancreas to make insulin

HOW DOES THE BODY CONTROL BLOOD SUGAR OR BLOOD GLUCOSE?

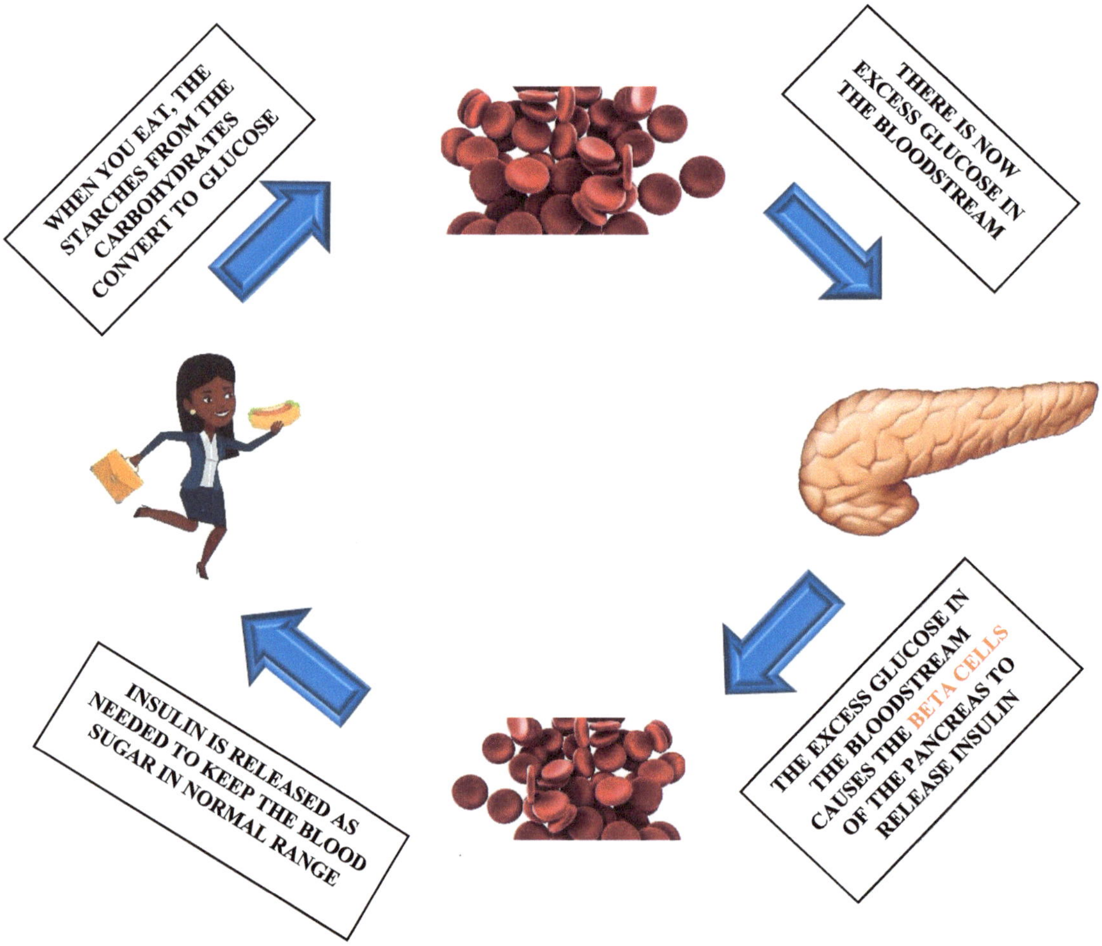

- WHEN YOU EAT, THE STARCHES FROM THE CARBOHYDRATES CONVERT TO GLUCOSE
- THERE IS NOW EXCESS GLUCOSE IN THE BLOODSTREAM
- THE EXCESS GLUCOSE IN THE BLOODSTREAM CAUSES THE BETA CELLS OF THE PANCREAS TO RELEASE INSULIN
- INSULIN IS RELEASED AS NEEDED TO KEEP THE BLOOD SUGAR IN NORMAL RANGE

TYPE I DIABETES: ALSO KNOWN AS INSULIN DEPENDENT DIABETES MELLITUS

A. Onset: Starts at childhood

B. You take insulin because your pancreas does not function **(The pancreas produces no insulin)**

C. 1st sign of Type I Diabetes is Diabetes Keto-Acidosis **(DKA)**

HOW DO YOU DEVELOP DKA?

The pancreas releases insulin to take the glucose out of the vascular space **(blood)** and brings the glucose into the cells. However, since the pancreas is unable to produce insulin, the glucose builds up in the vascular space **(blood)** and your cells are craving and starving for energy. The cells begin to breakdown fat and protein for energy. When fat is broken down, you get ketones **(acids)**. This places the patient into metabolic acidosis.

TYPE II DIABETES: ALSO KNOWN AS NON-INSULIN DEPENDENT DIABETES MELLITUS

A. The pancreas is functioning but not well

B. The pancreas produces too little or not enough insulin

C. These clients are typically overweight and are not producing enough insulin to maintain the glucose intake

HOW DOES THE CLIENT FIND OUT THAT HE/SHE HAS TYPE II DIABETES?

A. **Oops!!** they keep going back to the doctor for a wound that won't heal or frequent vaginal infections

   1. Why frequent vaginal infections? Bacteria gains strength in a high sugar environment

Treatment for Type II Diabetes

A. Diet & Exercise, *then*

B. Add Oral Agents, *then*

C. Add Insulin

Diabetes Signs & Symptoms

A. **Polyuria**: Excessive Urinating

B. **Polydipsia**: Excessive Thirst

C. **Polyphagia**: Excessive Eating

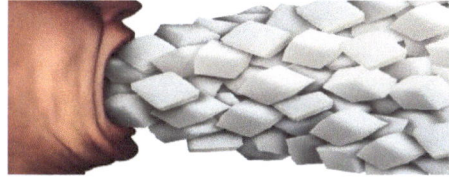

Scenario: The RN enters a diabetic client's room and they are unconscious. Will you treat this client as if they are hyperglycemic or hypoglycemic? and How will you provide treatment for this client?

Answer: Treat the client as hypoglycemic and give D50W (You need a angiocath/large bore IV & it is hard to push) or Injectable Glucagon (Use when there is no IV access & give IM)

Hypoglycemia Signs & Symptoms

A. Cold & Clammy Need Some Candy (Have the client eat a simple sugar)

   Once the blood sugar is up, have the client eat protein and a complex carbohydrate

B. Dizziness

C. Diaphoresis

COMPLICATIONS OF DIABETES

A. **DKA (Diabetic Ketoacidosis)**

   1. Increases in blood sugar can cause a client to develop illnesses and infections

   2. Usually the 1st sign of diabetes

   3. Associated with Type I Diabetes

   4. **Here is the rundown:**

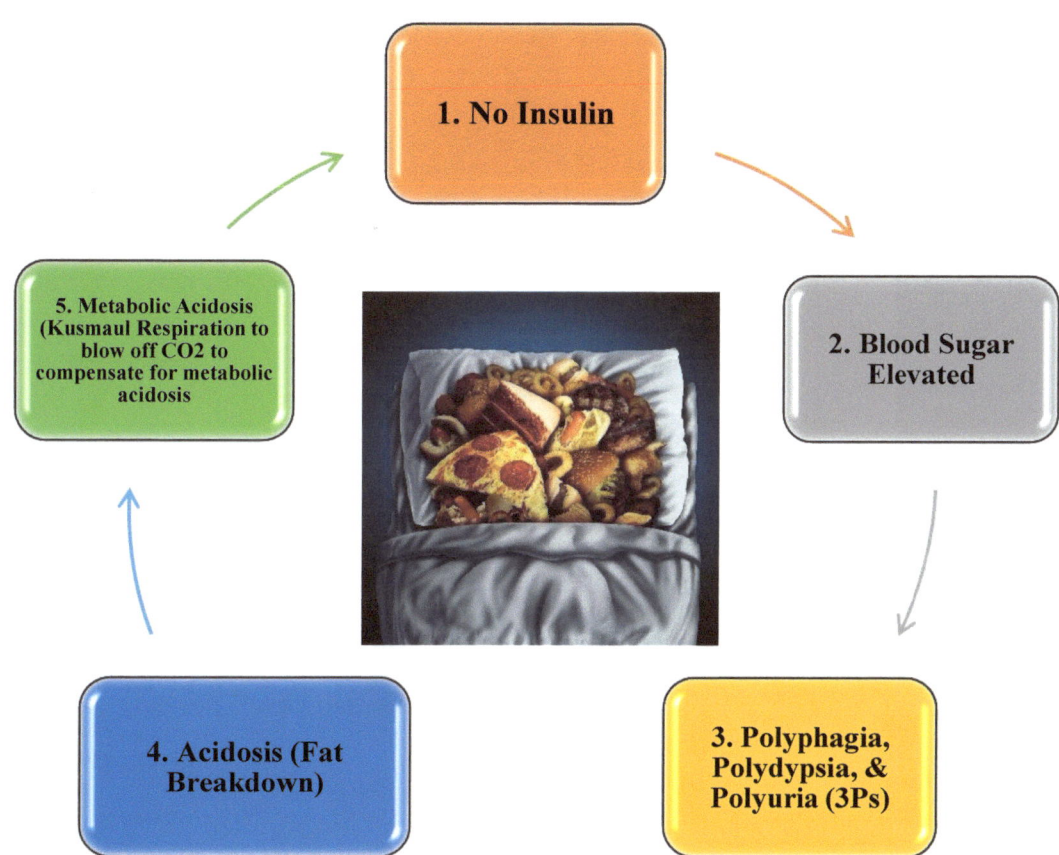

1. No Insulin
2. Blood Sugar Elevated
3. Polyphagia, Polydypsia, & Polyuria (3Ps)
4. Acidosis (Fat Breakdown)
5. Metabolic Acidosis (Kusmaul Respiration to blow off CO_2 to compensate for metabolic acidosis)

DKA TREATMENT

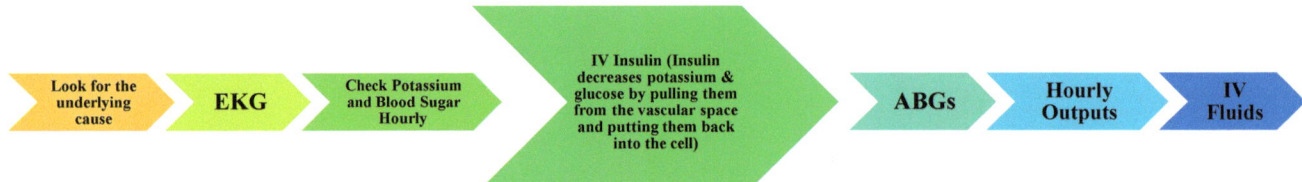

B. **Vascular Issues**

1. **Diabetic Retinopathy**: Diabetes complication that affects eyes. This is when high blood sugar levels cause damage to blood vessels in the retina.

2. **Diabetic Nephropathy**: Diabetic nephropathy is damage to your kidneys caused by diabetes. In severe cases, it can lead to kidney failure. However, not everyone with diabetes has kidney damage.

3. Poor circulation due to damage to the blood vessels (Uncontrolled blood sugar decreases the size of the vessel, thereby, blood flow decreases.

4. Neuropathy
    a. **Neurogenic Bladder**: Bladder does not empty completely
    b. **Gastroparesis**: Delayed stomach emptying, therefore high risk for aspiration
    c. **Foot & Leg Problems**: Numbness, pain, & paresthesia
    d. **Sexual Issues**: Decrease sensation & Impotence

5. Risk of Infection is High

C. HHNK (Hypertonic Hyperosmolar Non-Ketotic Coma)

1. This is associated with Type II Diabetes

2. It mimics DKA but there are no ketones (acidosis)

3. The pancreas is making just enough insulin so the client is not breaking down body fat

NO FAT = NO KETONES = NO ACIDOSIS

4. The client will not have kussmaul respirations

DIABETES AND TOOTH DECAY

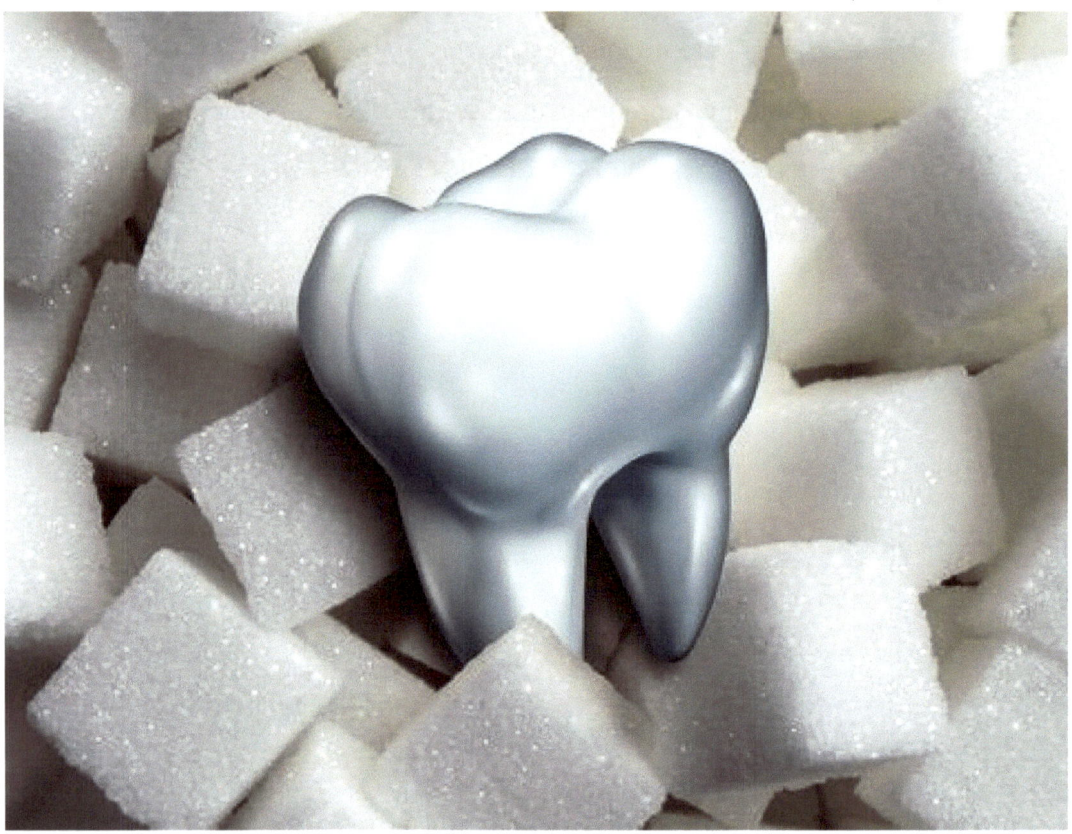

A. **Patients that have uncontrolled diabetes are at high risks for dental problems due to:**

    1. Infections of the gums and the bones that hold the teeth in place

    2. Reducing the blood supply to the gums

    3. Causes less saliva that allows for excess plaque buildup and tooth-decaying bacteria

B. **Signs and Symptoms**

    1. Have bad breath that will not go away

    2. Have sore or bleeding gums

    3. Get infections constantly

WHAT ABOUT MY THYROID?

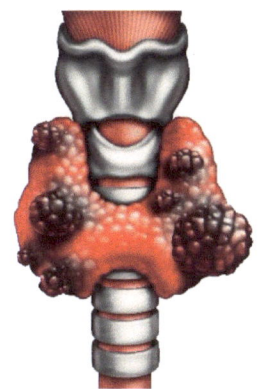

A. **Your thyroid produces three hormones: T3, T4, Calcitonin**

   1. Iodine is needed to make these hormones **(Eat Your Food!)**

   2. Your thyroid hormones give you energy!

B. **Hyperthyroid (Graves' Disease):** Way Too Much Energy!!

   1. **Signs & Symptoms**: Severe Weight Loss, Nervous, Exophthalmos, High Blood Pressure, Irritable, & T4 Level would be increased.

   2. **Treatment**:

      a. <u>**Iodine Medications**</u>: Potassium Iodide which is given in juice or milk with a straw

      b. <u>**Anti-Thyroids**</u>: Tapazole, PTU, and Propacil

         1. These medications stop the thyroid from producing thyroid hormones

         2. These medications have to be tapered and discontinued

      c. Beta Blockers such as Inderal **(Decreases Everything)**

         1. **INCREASED** Anxiety

         2. Heart Rate

         3. Blood Pressure

         4. Myocardial Contractility

         5. Will not release Epinephrine or Norepinephrine

         6. Mast the signs of hypoglycemia

d. One Dose of Radioactive Iodine (Tablet or Liquid Form)

  1. Destroys thyroid cells causing hypothyroidism

  2. Radioactive Precautions: Stay away from babies & No Kissing Anyone for 24 hours

  3. Rebound effect of post-radioactive iodine, the Nurse should look out for:

     THYROID STORM: It is associated with undertreated or untreated hyperthyroidism. It is **LIFE-THREATENING!!** During a thyroid storm, the patient's blood pressure, heart rate, and body temperature can rise to dangerously high levels.

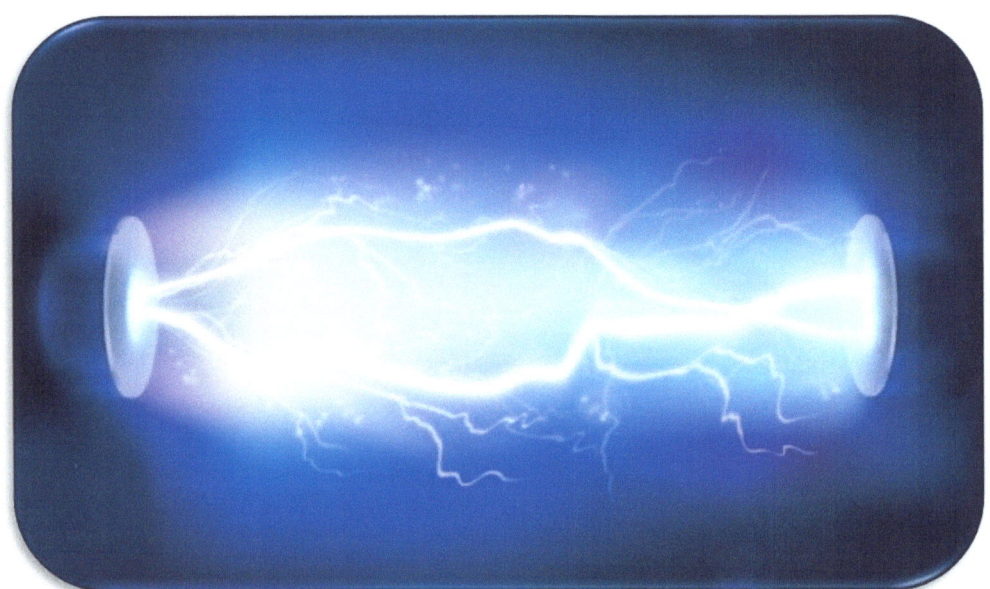

e. **Thyroidectomy (Complete/Partial):** Removal of all or part of the thyroid

  1. Post-Op Care

     a. Check for bleeding

     b. Put everything at arm's reach for the client

     c. Have a Trach Set at the bedside (Swelling, Recurrent laryngeal nerve damage, hypocalcemia)

     d. Assess for recurrent laryngeal nerve damage for hoarseness (This can lead to vocal cord paralysis causing airway obstruction which a trach will be placed)

     e. Teach the client how to support his/her neck

C. **Hypothyroid (Myxedema)**
   1. Absolutely NO ENERGY
   2. **Cretinism**: This is hypothyroidism that is present at birth. This is very dangerous and if left undetected, it can lead to slowed physical and mental development.
   3. **Signs & Symptoms**: Fatigue, Cold, No Expression, Weight Gain, & Slow GI
   4. **Treatment**:
      a. **Synthroid (Levothyroxine):** These clients stay on this medication for the rest of their lives
      b. Clients that have hypothyroidism usually have coronary artery disease
      c. When these clients start taking their medication, their energy level will increase

D. **Am I Paranoid, No It's Parathyroid**
   1. The parathyroid secretes parathyroid hormone (PTH). The PTH pulls calcium from the bones and places it in the blood. This causes the serum calcium level to **INCREASE**
      a. If you do not have any parathyroid hormone in the body, the serum calcium level will **DECREASE**
      b. If you have too much parathyroid hormone in your body, the serum calcium level will **INCREASE**
   2. Too much PTH causes serum calcium to go up and serum phosphorous to **DECREASE**

EQUATION: HYPERPARATHYROIDISM= HYPERCALCEMIA= HYPOPHOSPHATEMIA

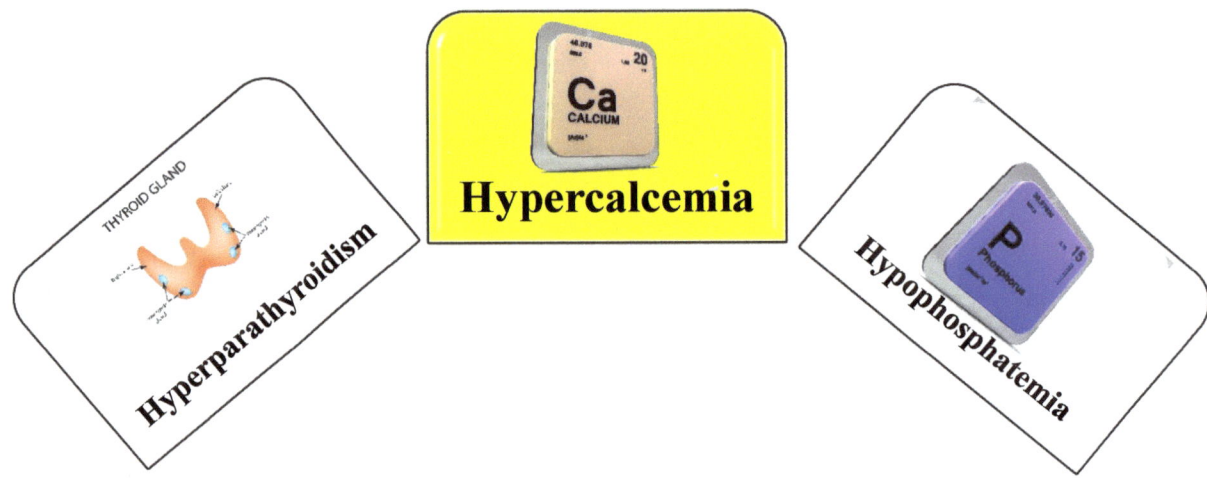

a. **Treatment**: Partial Parathyroidectomy (If you remove two of your parathyroid, your PTH secretion decreases)

3. Not enough PTH causes serum calcium to go down and serum phosphorous to go up

Equation: Hypoparathyroidism= Hypocalcemia= Hyperphosphatemia

a. **Treatment**:

1. Oral calcium carbonate tablets. Oral calcium supplements can increase calcium levels in your blood
2. Vitamin D: High doses of vitamin D can help your body absorb calcium and eliminate phosphorus
3. Foods Rich in Calcium: Dairy products, green leafy vegetables, and broccoli

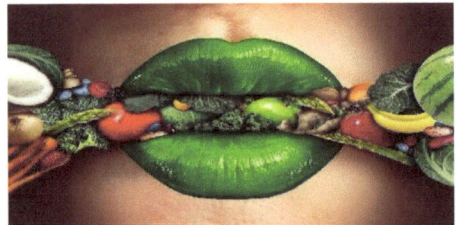

4. Foods Low in Phosphorous: avoid carbonated soft drinks (which contain phosphoric acid), limiting meats, hard cheeses, and whole grains

ADRENAL CORTEX ISSUES

A. **Addison's Disease:** NOT ENOUGH STEROIDS, HIGH POTASSIUM, & SHOCK

   1. Adrenocortical Insufficiency

   2. **Aldosterone** helps you to retain sodium and water and lose potassium. However, insufficiency causes the reverse, you will lose sodium and water and retain potassium

      a. If a client does not have enough mineralocorticoids, glucocorticoids, or sex hormones, then they are insufficient

   3. **Signs & Symptoms**

      a. Hyperkalemia: Muscle Twitching= weakness= flaccid paralysis because your serum K+ is high

      b. Hyperpigmentation

      c. Hypoglycemia

      d. Vitiligo (white patchy area of depigmented skin)

      e. Decrease bowel sounds

      f. Anorexia/nausea

      g. Hypotension

      If you run a urine or blood analysis on the client, their adrenocorticotropin hormones will be absent

   4. **Treatments**

      a. Will be placed on mineralocorticoid (must monitor weight while on medication)

      b. They will be losing weight

      c. Losing sodium and water (Combat Shock & Give Processed fruit juice/broth (lots of sodium))

B. **Cushing's Syndrome**: These clients can receive too many steroids and develop Cushing's Syndrome from <u>Exogenous administration</u>: When a person is taking steroids for treatment of COPD or asthma, organ transplants, autoimmune disorders, allergic responses, and chemotherapy. **(TOO MANY STEROIDS)**

1. Cushing's Disease can occur from the following: Pituitary adenoma increases secretion of ACTH, Bilaterally Adrenal Hyperplasia, Adrenal Carcinoma or Adenoma, and Malignancies.
2. These clients have too many glucocorticoids, sex hormones, and mineralocorticoids
    a. Too Many Mineralocorticoids
        1. Fluid Volume Excess (High Blood Pressure)
        2. Weight Gain

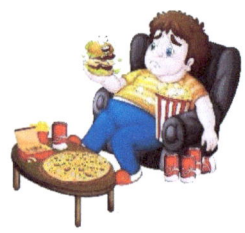

        3. CHF
        4. Truncal Obesity (redistribution of fat, lipogenesis)
        5. Moon Faced (fluid retention or gat redistribution)
        6. Buffalo hump (fat redistribution)
    b. Too Many Glucocorticoids
        1. Thin Extremities
        2. Increased Risk for Infection
        3. Growth Arrest
        4. Hyperglycemia
        5. Psychoses to Depression
    c. Too Many Sex
        1. Oily Acne/Skin
        2. Poor Sex Drive (High levels of adrenal steroids interfere with the ability of the pituitary gland to secrete FSH and LH and for the testes to make testosterone)
        3. Women with Male Traits

3. **Let's Take A Look At Some Pointers**

    a. If you performed a 24 hour urine of the client, the cortisol levels will be **HIGH**

    b. The serum K+ will be **LOW** due to the client will have too much mineralocorticoid (aldosterone).

4. **Treatment**

    a. Quiet Environment

    b. Adrenalectomy (Bilateral or Unilateral): If both are removed, they are on replacement therapy for life.

    c. Avoid Infection

    d. The Client Pre-Diet Treatment Will Contain: Increase in K+, Ca2+, Protein, & Decrease (Steroids Decrease Serum Ca2+ by Making You Excrete It Through The GI Tract)

    e. If you run a urinalysis on this Client, it will contain ketones and glucose

NCLEX PRACTICE QUESTIONS

1. The RN is observing another RN prepare to give a client in diabetic ketoacidosis 60 units of NPH insulin IV bolus. Which of the following interventions by the RN is appropriate?

    A. Instruct the RN to follow the NPH IV bolus with 10 to 15 units per hour in NS

    B. Tell the RN that only regular insulin may be administered IV

    C. Assist the RN in preparing the injection by rotating the vial of NPH insulin prior to drawing up the insulin

    D. Ask the RN to give the client the NPH insulin IV bolus for the experience

2. Which of the following should the RN include in the instructions given to a client with diabetes mellitus on how to prevent hypoglycemia?

    A. Have a family member learn to inject insulin if symptoms appear

    B. Ingest complex carbohydrates if symptoms appear

    C. Eat a snack or meal every four to five hours while awake

    D. Increase insulin if moderate exercise is planned

3. The RN should instruct a client with diabetes mellitus and the client's family about the clinical manifestations of DKA before discharge. Which of the following should be included? **SELECT ALL THAT APPLY**

    A. Shallow, labored respirations

    B. Tremors

    C. Dehydration

    D. Abdominal pain

    E. Acetone Breath

    F. Cold, clammy skin

4. Which of the following should be included in the assessment of a client with diabetes mellitus who is experiencing a hypoglycemic reaction? **SELECT ALL THAT APPLY**

   A. Nervousness

   B. Tremors

   C. Flushed skin

   D. Constricted Pupils

   E. Profuse perspiration

   F. Extreme thirst

5. The RN conducts a health hx for client with Type I diabetes mellitus. Which of the following client statements best describe the onset characteristics of this type of diabetes?

   A. My fasting blood sugars are always between 110 mg/dL and 126 mg/dL

   B. I was dx during the 5th month of my pregnancy

   C. When I hit 40, I began to notice I was urinating more frequently and picking up weight

   D. One day I passed out after I had terrible nausea, abdominal pain, and vomiting

6. The RN is admitting a client suspected of having Cushing's syndrome. Which of following assessments support the dx of Cushing's syndrome? **SELECT ALL THAT APPLY**

   A. HTN

   B. Hyperglycemia

   C. Fat pad accumulations above the clavicles

   D. Hyperpigmentation of the skin on the abdomen and breasts

   E. Decreased facial hair and body

   F. Slender trunk with enlarged legs and arms

7. The diet for a client with hypoparathyroidism should be high in calcium and low in phosphorus. The RN instructs the client to eat which of the following foods?

    A. Cauliflower

    B. Milk

    C. Green leafy vegetables

    D. Cheese

8. The post-op orders for a client who has had the parathyroid gland removed include using Chvostek's sign to assess for signs of tetany. Which of the following is the appropriate assessment technique the RN should implement?

    A. Tap sharply over the facial nerves

    B. Occlude the blood flow in the wrist

    C. Listen for a crowing sound with inspirations

    D. Observe respiratory depth and rate

9. The RN is caring for a client with myxedema. Which of the following would indicate to the RN that the client's condition is deteriorating?

    A. Episodes of chills and cold skin

    B. Difficulty in arousing the client for medications

    C. An increase in respirations and pulse rate

    D. Client complaints of palpitations

10. The RN develops a plan of care for the immediate post-op period for a client who had a thyroidectomy. The plan should include measures to:

    A. Administer medications to decrease vascularity of the thyroid glands

    B. Correct fluid and electrolyte balance

    C. Prevent complications of respiratory obstruction

    D. Promote range-of-motion exercise to the neck

11. Which of the following client statements should the RN report to the MD prior to scheduling a radioactive iodine uptake and excretion test?

    A. My husband and I are vegetarians

    B. I've been taking over-the-counter cough medicine for the past two weeks

    C. I take a baby aspirin every day since my heart attack last year

    D. We like to drink a glass of wine with our meals

12. The RN should report which of the following client assessments as consistent with a dx of Graves' Disease? **SELECT ALL THAT APPLY**

    A. Exophthalmos

    B. Weight loss

    C. Bradycardia

    D. Lethargy

    E. Heat intolerance

    F. Cold, clammy skin

NCLEX ANSWERS

1.) **B**
   Rationale: Only regular insulin, which is clear, can be administered IV

2.) **C**
   Rationale: Meals or snacks every four to five hours while awake will maintain consistent blood sugar levels and should aid in the prevention of hypoglycemia

3.) **C, D, E**
   Rationale: In DKA, the body burns fats, which in turns increases the amount of ketone bodies. An increase in ketone bodies causes acetone breath, which has a fruity odor. DKA is a state of hyperglycemia

4.) **A, B, E**
Rationale: In hypoglycemia, the blood glucose levels fall, resulting in sympathetic nervous system responses such as tremors, sweating, and nervousness

5.) **D**
Rationale: Type I Diabetes has an acute onset with nausea, abdominal pain, and vomiting and is often dx after the client becomes comatose with ketoacidosis

6.) **A, B, C**
Rationale: Cushing's syndrome is an overproduction of glucocorticoids and androgens from the adrenal cortex. These hormones produce fat pad accumulations, a buffalo hump in the neck, and supraclavicular areas. Hyperglycemia and HTN are also clinical manifestations

7.) **C**

Rationale: Green leafy vegetables are high in calcium and low in phosphorus. Milk and cheese products are high in calcium but also high in phosphorus

8.) **A**

Rationale: Tetany is neuromuscular irritability characterized by spasms and tremors. Chvostek's sign is performed by tapping sharply over the facial nerves and is positive if is causes spasms and twitching in the region of the nose, mouth, and eyes

9.) **B**

Rationale: The most life-threatening complication for the client with myxedema is myxedema coma. If a client with myxedema becomes unable to be aroused, the client is progressing into a coma

10.) **C**

   Rationale: **A thyroidectomy is the removal of the thyroid gland through a neck incision. Immediately post-op there is the potential complication of airway obstruction by edema formation**

11.) **B:**

   Rationale: **Medications and foods containing iodine alter the results of radioactive iodine tests. Over-the-counter medicines contain iodine**

12.) **A, B, E**

   Rationale: **Hyperthyroidism (Graves' Disease) is characterized by an increase in the metabolic rate, an accumulation of fluid in the fat pads behind the eyes, and protruding eyeballs (exophthalmos). The client also experiences hyperexcitability, heat intolerance, nervousness, and weight loss despite increased appetite**

REFERENCES

Berkowitz, A. (2007). *Clinical pathophysiology made ridiculously simple*. Miami, FL: MedMaster Inc.

Ignatavicius, D., & Workman, M. (2006). *Medical-Surgical Nursing critical thinking for collaborative care*. Saint Louis, Missouri: Elsevier Saunders.

PHOTO CREDITS

http://www.dreamstime.com